The CMS Restraint
Training Requirements
Handbook

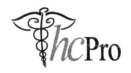

The CMS Restraint Training Requirements Handbook is published by HCPro, Inc.

Copyright © 2007 HCPro, Inc.

All rights reserved. Printed in the United States of America.   5   4   3   2   1

ISBN 978-1-60146-068-4

HCPro, Inc., provides information resources for the healthcare industry.

HCPro, Inc., is not affiliated in any way with The Joint Commission, which owns the JCAHO and Joint Commission trademarks.

Jay Kumar, Editor
Brian Driscoll, Executive Editor
John Novack, Group Publisher
Janell Lukac, Layout Artist
Sada Preisch, Proofreader
Darren Kelly, Books Production Supervisor
Susan Darbyshire, Art Director
Claire Cloutier, Production Manager
Jean St. Pierre, Director of Operations

Advice given is general. Readers should consult professional counsel for specific legal, ethical, or clinical questions.

Arrangements can be made for quantity discounts. For more information, contact:
HCPro, Inc.
P.O. Box 1168
Marblehead, MA 01945
Telephone: 800/650-6787 or 781/639-1872
Fax: 781/639-2982
E-mail: *customerservice@hcpro.com*

Visit HCPro at its World Wide Web sites:
www.hcpro.com **and** *www.hcmarketplace.com*

6/2007
21224

Contents

The CMS Restraint Training Requirements **Handbook**

Introduction

In January 2007, new patients' rights regulations from the Centers for Medicare & Medicaid Services (CMS) went into effect, requiring hospitals to rewrite their policies about restraint and seclusion. The new regulations in the *Conditions of Participation (CoP)* set forth, among other things, new training requirements.

There are five sections to the patients' rights standards. The first four sections were published without making any changes to the current *CoP*. The fifth section includes the patient's right to be free from unnecessary restraint and seclusion. This section combined two separate sections on medical and surgical restraints and behavioral health restraints. It includes 16 rules on restraint and seclusion, covering:

- Freedom from restraint and seclusion
- Less restrictive interventions
- Orders
- Notification
- Care plans

- Discontinuation

- Assessment and reassessment

- Performance improvement

- Use

- Time limits

- Renewal

- Staff education

- Monitoring

- Death protocol

It's important to understand that the core definition of *restraint* remains essentially the same, with the distinction between the more restrictive time limitations clarified, not changed. The new definition says a restraint is any manual method, physical or mechanical device, material, or equipment that immobilizes or reduces the ability of a patient to move his or her arms, legs, body, or head freely. It also includes a drug or medication when it is used as a restriction to manage the patient's behavior or restrict the patient's freedom of movement and is not a standard treatment or dosage for the patient's condition. The CMS says all patients have the right to be free from physical or mental abuse and corporal punishment. All patients have the right to be free from restraint or seclusion, of any form, imposed as a means of coercion, discipline, convenience, or retaliation by staff. Restraint or seclusion may only be imposed to ensure the immediate physical safety of the patient, a staff member, or others, and must be discontinued at the earliest possible time.

A restraint does *not* include devices—such as orthopedically prescribed devices, surgical dressings or bandages, protective helmets, or other methods that involve the physical holding of a patient for the purpose of:

- Conducting routine physical examinations or tests
- Permitting the patient to participate in activities without the risk of physical harm (this does not include a physical escort)

The definition of *seclusion*—the involuntary confinement of a person in a room or area in which the person is physically prevented from leaving—did not change.

Those who provide staff training on restraint and seclusion use must be qualified as evidenced by education, training, and experience in techniques used to address patient behaviors, according to the new regulations. All direct care staff must receive training in the hospital's restraint and seclusion policies and approaches, and all staff who may be involved in the use of restraint must be trained in safe use of restraint, including the use of mechanical restraint devices, takedowns, and holding.

Hospital leadership sets the standards for the current restraint and seclusion policies (medical/surgical and behavioral). The policies should set clear expectations for a safe environment in which restraint and seclusion are used only as a last resort. Staff is expected to commit to minimizing the factors that might result in the need to restrain or seclude a patient.

The new training requirements

The patient has the right to safe implementation of restraint or seclusion by trained staff. You must be able to demonstrate competency in the application of restraints, implementation of seclusion, monitoring, assessment, and providing care for a patient in restraint or seclusion. Training should take place before staff perform any of the actions specified in the training requirements, as part of orientation, and subsequently on a periodic basis consistent with hospital policy.

Individuals providing staff training must be qualified as evidenced by education, training, and experience in techniques used to address patient behavior. The hospital must document in staff personnel records that the training and demonstration of competency were successfully completed.

The new regulations spell out the following restraint and seclusion training requirements for staff:

Safe application of restraints

You should be able to demonstrate and ensure that when you select a type of restraint, you take the following steps:

- Select the proper size for the patient's weight.
- Note "front" and "back" of the restraint and apply correctly.
- Pad any bony prominences.
- Use a knot that can easily be released (half-bow).
- Secure restraints to the bed springs or frame, never to the mattress or bed rails. When an adjustable bed is in use, secure the restraints to the parts of the bed that move with the patient. Never secure a restraint to a bed rail or mattress.
- Adjust restraint to maintain good body alignment, comfort, and safety.
- Ensure restraints are not too tight. (Test to be certain you can insert two fingers in between restraint and skin.)

Implementation of seclusion

You need to demonstrate knowledge of the definition of seclusion, which is the involuntary confinement of a person alone in a room or an area where the person is physically prevented from leaving. Seclusion does not include confinement on a locked unit or ward where the patient is with others. Seclusion may only be used for the management of violent or self-destructive behavior. Seclusion is seldom used in general healthcare settings.

Monitoring of patients in restraint/seclusion

You must be able to discuss the monitoring of a patient in restraints. The condition of the patient who is restrained or secluded must be monitored by a physician, other licensed independent practitioner, or trained staff that have completed the CMS training requirements.

This monitoring includes:

- Ensuring the physical and emotional well-being of the patient

- Maintaining the patient's rights, dignity, and safety

- Documenting the type, location, and proper application of the restraining device(s)

- Documented at least once per shift and when changed

- Assessing the rationale for restraint on an ongoing basis

- Documented at least once per shift (observed condition or behavior)

- Considering alternatives to and less restrictive forms of restraint

- Documented at least once per shift

- Completing other monitoring activities based on the currently approved medical restraint form

- Documented per policy

Assessment of patients in restraint/seclusion

You should conduct an initial assessment of a patient at the time of the patient's admission to determine if restraint is necessary. The assessment should include the following:

- Consideration of medical conditions or disability that might increase the risk of harm to the patient during a restraint episode

- Any history of sexual or physical abuse that might increase the risk to the patient during restraint

- Documentation that the patient—and, if appropriate, the patient's family—was informed of the organization's philosophy regarding use of restraint or seclusion

You must, when appropriate, discuss the role of the family in relation to restraint with the patient and family. You must also determine whether the patient has a mental health advance directive, which should indicate the patient's preference for treatment in case the patient becomes dangerous to him or herself or others. If the patient has an advance directive, the hospital must provide the information to staff.

When restraint or seclusion is used for the management of violent or self-destructive behavior that jeopardizes the immediate physical safety of the patient, a staff member, or others, the patient must be seen face-to-face within one hour after the initiation of the intervention. The patient may be assessed by a physician or other licensed independent practitioner (LIP), or a registered nurse or physician assistant who has been trained in the CMS restraint and seclusion training requirements. Check to see if your state has stricter requirements.

If the face-to-face evaluation is conducted by a trained registered nurse or physician assistant, that individual must consult the attending physician or other LIP who is responsible for the patient's care as soon as possible after the completion of the one-hour face-to-face evaluation.

Simultaneous restraint and seclusion use is only permitted if the patient is continually monitored face-to-face by an assigned, trained staff member or by trained staff using both video and audio equipment.

Staff authorized to carry out restraint must be trained to measure vital signs and know the relevance of vital signs to restrained patients. They must be able to recognize and respond to needs for nutrition and hydration, proper circulation and movement of limbs, and hygiene and elimination.

Providing care for a patient in restraint or seclusion

You should modify the patient's written plan of care to indicate the type of restraint and the goals of the restraint use.

Techniques to identify triggers of circumstances that require use of restraint or seclusion

You should watch for the following indications to consider using restraint or seclusion when less restrictive means would not be effective in protecting the patient:

- The patient is pulling at tubes, lines, or dressings
- The confused patient is interfering with the provision of care
- The patient's actions are endangering him or herself: for example, if the patient is thrashing around in bed or attempting to get out of bed in a way or under conditions where it might cause harm (including when such behavior is related to acute withdrawal syndrome)
- The patient's diagnosis or condition is such that he or she may unpredictably and suddenly awaken and harm him or herself; e.g., a) when an intubated patient is being weaned from propofol or b) when an intubated patient has a neurological condition that may cause him or her to unpredictably and suddenly awaken with a significant risk of self-extubation before staff have an opportunity to intervene

Use of nonphysical intervention skills

You should be well-versed in the use of nonphysical intervention skills such as verbal and nonverbal communication, reduced stimulation, active listening, diversionary techniques, limit setting, and as-needed (PRN) medication.

Choosing the least restrictive intervention

Restraint should not be used when less restrictive interventions would be effective. These include environmental techniques such as:

- Designing the clinical unit to avoid patient crowding and provide some settings where patients can be by themselves to calm down

- Providing easy access to staff and facilitation of conversation with staff as a means of blowing off steam or getting advice

- Access to activities that will either preoccupy the patient's attention or use up physical energy (e.g., interesting videos or exercise equipment)

Another type of less restrictive intervention consists of steps that staff should take on the spot when it appears an individual is about to go into crisis. These steps are generally called de-escalation and are heavily dependent on proper staff training to recognize the situation and deal with it.

Safe application and use of all types of restraint and seclusion used in facility

You must consider the following information when selecting the type of restraint you will use:

- The patient's expressed preference provided at admission in the advance directive

- The initial assessment, which contains the patient's history, physical strength and limitations, and vulnerabilities

- The dimensions of the emergency that the restraint is intended to end

You should receive training in how to recognize and respond to signs of physical and psychological distress (e.g., positional asphyxia). Among the restraint options a hospital might consider having available are four-point leather restraints, two-point restraints, Posey vests, and seclusion. You need to be able to demonstrate and follow the manufacturer's directions when applying restraints.

Clinical identification of specific behavioral changes that indicate restraint is no longer needed

You must discontinue the restraint when the behavior or condition that was the basis for the restraint order is resolved, regardless of the duration of the enabling order. You should be able to recognize the behavioral criteria for discontinuation of restraint and assist patients in meeting these criteria. If you are not permitted to make the decision to discontinue restraint, you must call supervisory staff, who will then make the decision to release.

Monitoring physical well-being of patient

Continuous, in-person observation:

- Monitoring of patients in restraint or seclusion is done through continuous in-person observation by a competent staff member

  Exception: After the first hour, a patient in seclusion *without restraint* may be continuously monitored using simultaneous video and audio equipment, if consistent with the patient's condition and wishes

- If the patient is on a physical hold, a second staff person shall be assigned to observe the patient

Monitoring:

- You should assess the patient at the initiation of restraint or seclusion and every 15 minutes thereafter

- The assessment should include the following, unless it is inappropriate for the type of restraint or seclusion employed:

  - Signs of any injury associated with applying restraint or seclusion

  - Nutrition and hydration

  - Circulation and range of motion in the extremities

  - Vital signs

  - Hygiene and elimination

  - Physical and psychological status and comfort

  - Readiness for discontinuation of restraint or seclusion

Use of first aid techniques and certification in CPR use

You should be able to demonstrate competency in the use of first-aid techniques and certification in the use of cardiopulmonary resuscitation, including required periodic recertification. The sample competency forms on the next few pages will help you develop your own competencies.

Sample competency form 1

Application of restraints		
Name: _____ **Date:** _____		
Skill: Restraints, application of _____		

Steps	Completed	Comments
1. Verbalizes need to assess patients requiring restraints and identifies alternative to restraints		
2. Identifies nurse's and physician's roles in application of restraints		
3. Describes time frame for patient assessment/ documentation		
4. Documents restraints on restraint log		
5. Chest restraint a. Applies chest restraint and adjusts waist belt to fit b. Demonstrates how to secure to bedspring frame (not side rails) or back frame of wheelchair		

6. Soft restraints
 	
  a. Verbalizes criteria for application of restraints to extremities (single restraint, wrists only, all extremities)
 	
  b. Applies soft restraint to extremity		

7. Mitt restraints a. Applies mitt restraint		
8. Leather restraints a. Verbalizes role of personnel in applying leather restraints		

Self-assessment	Evaluation/validation methods	Levels	Type of validation	Comments
❑ Experienced ❑ Need practice ❑ Never done ❑ Not applicable (based on scope of practice)	❑ Verbal ❑ Demonstration/observation ❑ Practical exercise ❑ Interactive class	❑ Beginner ❑ Intermediate ❑ Expert	❑ Orientation ❑ Annual ❑ Other	

_____   _____
Employee signature   *Observer signature*

Sample competency form 2

Restraints (role of nursing assistant)		
Name: _____ **Date:** _____		
Skill: Restraints (role of nursing assistant) _____		

Steps	Completed	Comments
1. Verbalizes nursing assistant's role in safety evaluation of restraints		
2. States how and where to document restraints		
3. Soft restraints: a. Demonstrates how to remove and reapply soft restraints to extremities b. Demonstrates how to secure to bedspring frame (not side rails) using slipknot		
4. Mitt restraints: a. Demonstrates how to remove and reapply unit restraints		
5. Leather restraints (optional): a. Demonstrates how to remove and reapply leather restraints		

6. Verbalizes comprehension
   and support of nursing two-
   hour assessment of patient's
   restraints

Self-assessment	Evaluation/ validation methods	Levels	Type of validation	Comments
❏ Experienced ❏ Need practice ❏ Never done ❏ Not applicable (based on scope of practice)	❏ Verbal ❏ Demonstra-tion/ observa-tion ❏ Practical exercise ❏ Interactive class	❏ Beginner ❏ Intermediate ❏ Expert	❏ Orienta-tion ❏ Annual ❏ Other	

Employee signature   *Observer signature*

Sample competency form 3

Seclusion restraint (behavioral health)		
Name: _____ Date: _____		
Skill: Seclusion restraint (behavioral health) _____		
Steps	**Completed**	**Comments**
Initiation of seclusion 1. Team of three or more staff and RN leader formed using principles of nonviolent crisis intervention.		
2. Leader informs patient of reason for restraints/seclusion and behaviors that must be exhibited to be released from seclusion.		
Leader directs team members and communicates with patient.		
4. When in room, patient is searched, street clothes and dangerous objects are removed, and patient is placed in a hospital gown.		

5. Vital signs obtained and documented. If team is unable to obtain vital signs due to patient's condition, documentation states reason for failure to obtain vital signs.		
6. Patient placed on mattress in seclusion room.		
7. Staff members exit the room one at a time.		
8. After patient secluded, staff critiques process (postvention).		
Documentation on seclusion/ restraint log and orders 1. Documents patient's behavior leading to necessity of restraint/seclusion.		
2. Documents less restrictive means/alternatives to restraint/seclusion tried prior to seclusion.		
3. Discusses need for restraint/ seclusion with patient/family and documents it.		

4. Obtains physician order with clinical justification for restraints/seclusion within one hour of implementation of seclusion.		
5. Written order time-limited and does not exceed four hours.		
6. Initiates TV and audio monitoring and informs patient.		
7. Documents patient assessment and has RN sign q 2h to determine if seclusion can be discontinued.		
8. Assesses patient's mental status and physical needs q 15 minutes and documents it in log.		

Self-assessment	Evaluation/validation methods	Levels	Type of validation	Comments
❏ Experienced ❏ Need practice ❏ Never done ❏ Not applicable (based on scope of practice)	❏ Verbal ❏ Demonstration/ observation ❏ Practical exercise ❏ Interactive class	❏ Beginner ❏ Intermediate ❏ Expert	❏ Orientation ❏ Annual ❏ Other	

_____   _____
Employee signature   *Observer signature*

Quiz

1. How many sections of the Centers for Medicare & Medicaid Services' (CMS) Patient Rights Conditions of Participation (CoP) were changed in January 2007?

2. What is not included in the official CMS definition of restraint?

3. True or false: Seclusion includes confinement on a locked unit or ward where the patient is with others.

4. How often should you document the type, location, and proper application of the restraining device?

5. How long after restraint or seclusion is used must the patient be assessed?

6. Provide six examples of nonphysical intervention skills.

7. True or false: Less restrictive interventions do no include environmental techniques.

8. What should the initial assessment contain?

9. True or false: The restraint must be discontinued when the patient's behavior or condition that was the basis for the restraint order is resolved, regardless of the duration of the order.

10. After how long is it acceptable to monitor a patient in seclusion without restraint by using video and audio equipment?

Answer key

1. One section was changed. The first four sections of the Patient Rights CoP were published without making any changes to the current CoP. The fifth section includes the changes to the restraint and seclusion requirements.

2. The revised CMS definition of restraint does not include devices—such as orthopedically prescribed devices, surgical dressings or badges, protective helmets, or other methods that involve the physical holding of a patient for the purpose of:

   • Conducting routine physical examinations or tests

   • Protecting the patient from falling out of bed

   • Permitting the patient to participate in activities without the risk of physical harm (this does not include a physical escort)

3. False.

4. At least once per shift and when changed.

5. The patient must be seen face-to-face within one hour after the initiation of the intervention.

6. Nonphysical intervention skills include verbal and non-verbal communication, reduced stimulation, active listening, diversionary techniques, limit setting, and as-needed medication.

7. False.

8. The patient's history, physical strength and limitations, and vulnerabilities.

9. True.

10. After the first hour, a patient in seclusion without restraint may be continuously monitored using simultaneous video and audio equipment, if consistent with the patient's condition and wishes.

CERTIFICATE OF COMPLETION

This is to certify that

_____

has read and successfully passed the final exam of

The CMS Restraint Training Requirements Handbook

_____

Robert Stuart
Senior Vice President/Chief Operating Officer